KETO BREAKFAST

Discover 30 Easy to Follow Ketogenic Breakfast Cookbook recipes for Your Low-Carb Diet with Gluten-Free and wheat to Maximize your weight loss

STEPHANIE BAKER

Copyright © Stephanie Baker

All rights reserved. No part of this book may be reproduced, scanned or distributed in any printed or electronic form without permission. Please do not participate in or encourage piracy of copyrighted materials in violation of the author's rights. Purchase only authorized editions.

1
COCONUT CURD AND FRAMBOISE

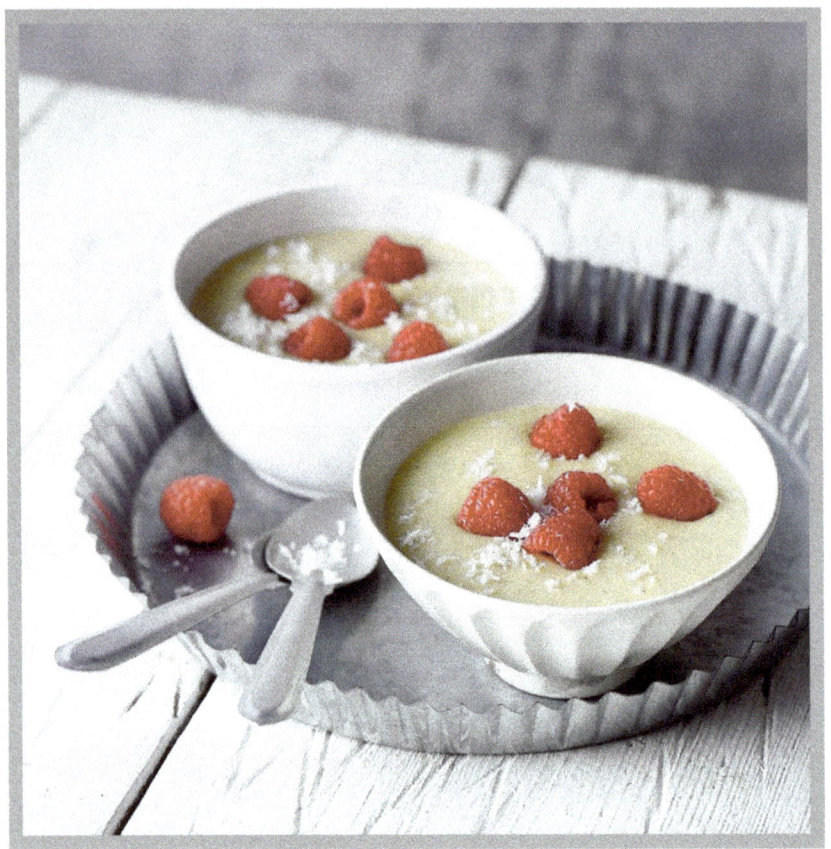

90 min.

525 kcal

Lightning

Serving 2

. . .

INGREDIENTS

- 200 g (canned) coconut milk
- 4 Eggs (M)
- 1 Pinch of powdered psyllium husk
- 2 Tbsp coconut meal
- 1/2 tablespoon of vanilla ground
- 1/2 teaspoon powdered cinnamon
- Seasoning
- 4 Ice-cold Butter Teaspoons
- 100 G of framboise

- 1 cup of dried coconut

PREPARATION

1. Place coconut milk , eggs, and psyllium husk powder in a heat-resistant bowl (made of metal if possible) with 100 ml warm water and mix quickly with the whisk until smooth. Stir in a smooth mixture and add coconut flour, cocoa, cinnamon and a pinch of salt.

1. Fill up enough pot with water for the water bath

about 1 cm high, and bring the water to a boil. Over the water bath heat the coconut and egg mixture in the bowl without it coming into contact with water. Constantly swirl the mixture for 10-12 minutes, so it doesn't flocculate. Remove until thick, and begin to thicken. This is easily detected when stirring through the increasing resistance.

1. Remove the coconut and egg mixture from the water bath immediately, whisk in the ice-cold butter until it has melted and spread the curd between two bowls of muesli. Cover for at least 6 hours, or better overnight, with cling film and chill. The curd gets a pudding-like consistency when cold.
2. Carefully wash the raspberries, pat dry, spread over the cream and garnish with desiccated coconut.
3. The curd with the same amount of blueberries or papaya, is also delicious. There is nothing wrong with the frozen goods as well. Put the fruit in a bowl to thaw the evening before, and put it in the fridge if you want it to be particularly fast in the morning.

2
FILLED OMELETTE WITH CHEESE

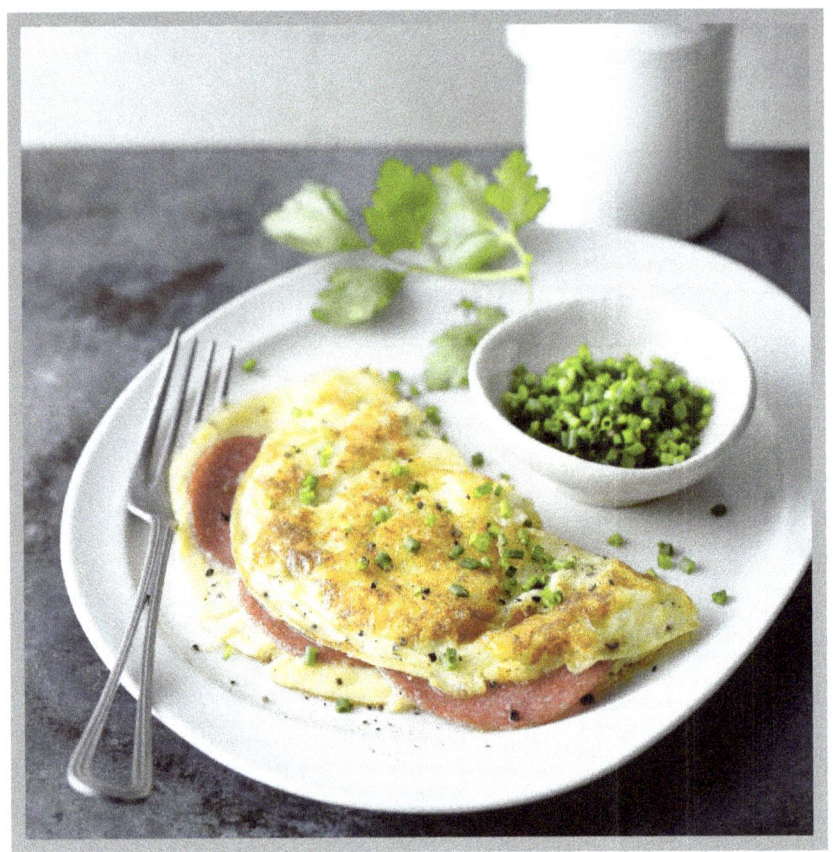

30 min.

400 kcal

Lightning

Serving 2

. . .

INGREDIENTS

- Gouda 50 g
- 50 g Cheese with parmesan
- 3 Owls (M)
- 2 cups of heavy cream
- Seasoning
- Pepper
- 2 Butter Teaspoons
- 4 Chives sticks
- 6 Salami slices
- 2 Cilantro-stalks

PREPARATION

1. Apply the Gouda and Parmesan coarsely, and combine well. Whisk the eggs and cream with a fork, and add salt and pepper to season.

1. Heat up 1 Teaspoon Butter over medium heat in a non-stick pan. Lay half of the cheese mixture evenly flat in the oven, and let the cheese melt for around 1 minute in the covered plate.
2. Place half of the egg mixture on top of the cheese in the saucepan and whisk to be spread. Cover the pan,

and bake the egg mixture for around 2 minutes over medium heat. Wash the chives, dry-shake, and cut into rolls.

1. Fill one half of the omelet with 3 slices of salami and use a spatula to carefully fold over the other half. Once again cover the pan and bake the omelet for 2 minutes. Flip the omelet and bake the other side for 2 minutes, until the mixture has thickened completely.

1. Flip the omelet onto a tray, keeping it warm and lined with foil. Bake the second omelet with the ingredients left over. Sprinkle with chives on both omelets and serve with coriander garnish.
2. Such ingredients as a filling on the breakfast board include plenty of variety: cheeses such as cream cheese, feta, mozzarella or a little crème fraîche, sliced vegetables such as cherry tomatoes, shallots, red onions, or peppers. On top of that, sweet, fresh herbs like basil, oregano, flat-leaf parsley, thyme or sage. Is there any leftover smoked ham in the fridge, Parma ham, smoked turkey breast or even breakfast bacon? Okay, just bring it in an omelet always.

HEARTY BREAD WITH ALMONDS

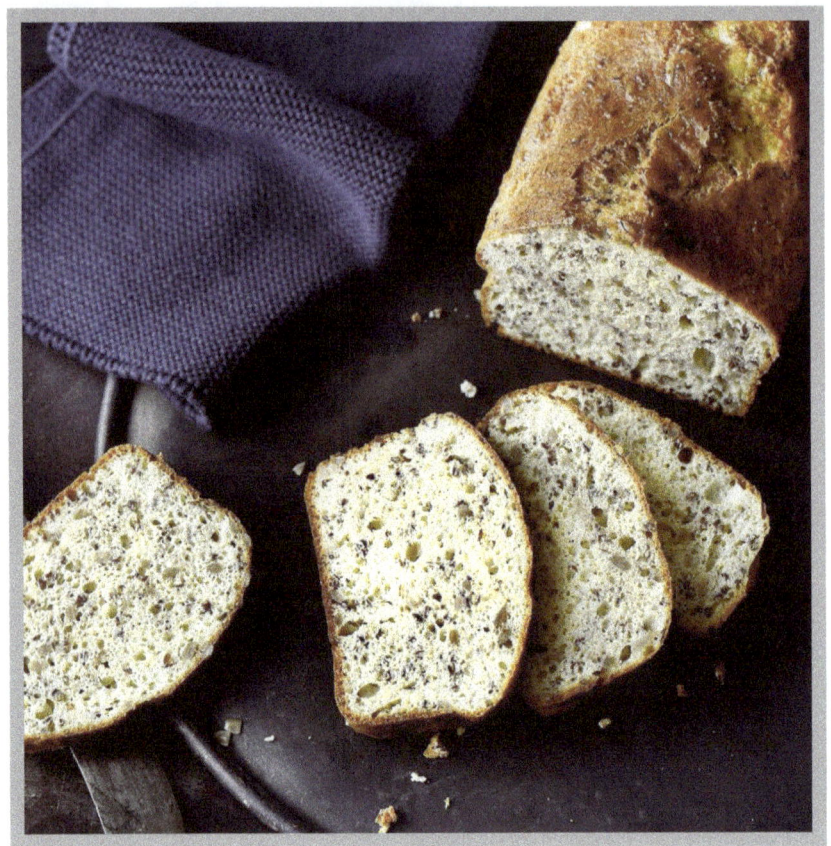

90 minutes

130 kcal

Lightning

Serving Dimensions

For 1 bread (roughly 15 slices)

INGREDIENTS

- Greek yogurt: 250 g
- 6 Owls (M)
- Seasoning
- 40 g Crushed linseed
- Sunflower seeds 50 g
- 120 grams of ground almonds
- 2 Tbsp powdered psyllium husk
- 2 Tbsp of baked soda
- Including:
- 1 Bread of the loaf
- Coconut oil to grease

PREPARATION

1. Oven preheat to 180 °. Grease coconut oil into the loaf tub. In a cup, mix yogurt, eggs and a pinch of salt, until smooth. Then add the seeds of the flax, the seeds of the sunflower and the almonds.
2. Add psyllium husk powder and baking powder and easily mix in with a whisk. Let the dough swell for 10 minutes, then fill the greased loaf pan and place in the middle of the oven.

1. Bake the batter for 45 minutes. Try taking it out, let it cool down briefly and turn the bread out of the pan with care. Let it cool off on a wire rack.

1. Offer the dough a distinctive taste that can vary again and again. Because that is z. B. Seeds from fennel, caraway seeds, dried thyme or rosemary.1 tsp is enough growing. A splash of red vinegar adds a good acidity to the crust.

BLUEBERRY BANANA PANCAKES WITH COCONUT

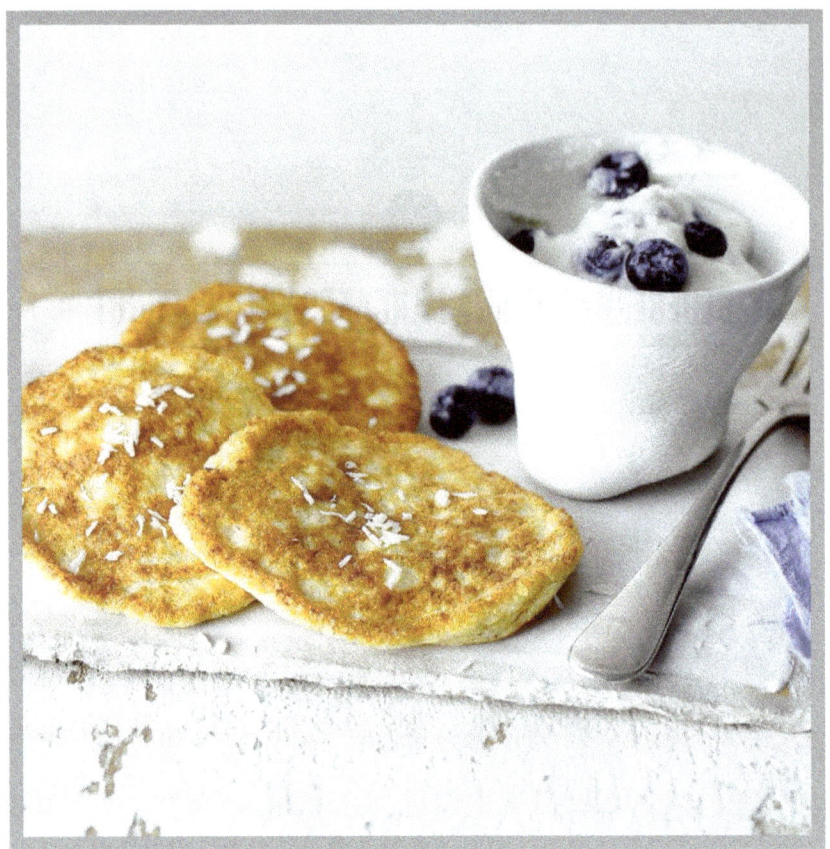

30 min.

Kcal 635

Lightning

Serving 2

. . .

INGREDIENTS

- 3 Owls (M)
- 80 g Fresh Cream
- 2 Tbsp of desiccated cocoa
- 2 Teaspoons of husk powder with psyllium
- 3 Tbsp olive oil
- To the yoghurt:
- 50 g Brownishes
- 200 g and yogurt
- 1 cup of coconut butter
- 1/2 tablespoon of vanilla ground
- Sugar with birch (xylitol, to taste)

PREPARATION

1. To form a smooth dough, mix the eggs, crème fraîche, desiccated coconut and psyllium husk powder quickly with a whisk. On. Let take 10 minutes to soak.

1. Alternatively, wash the yoghurt blueberries, drain them, and mash them a little with a fork. Stir and chill, add yogurt, coconut butter and ground vanilla. Where appropriate, season with birch sugar.

1. The coconut oil is heated in a large non-stick oven. Put 1-2 spoonfuls of batter per pancake in the pan and bake for approx. 2 Minutes over medium heat until golden brown on the underside. Turn on and brown for 1-2 minutes on the other side.

1. Bake eight pancakes in total, arrange on plates and serve with the blueberry yoghurt.

1. How everybody likes it. Before the evening the pancakes are easy to prepare and the next morning taste cold too. You can bake them fresh in the morning or warm them up briefly in the microwave or oven if you don't like that.

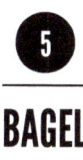

BAGEL

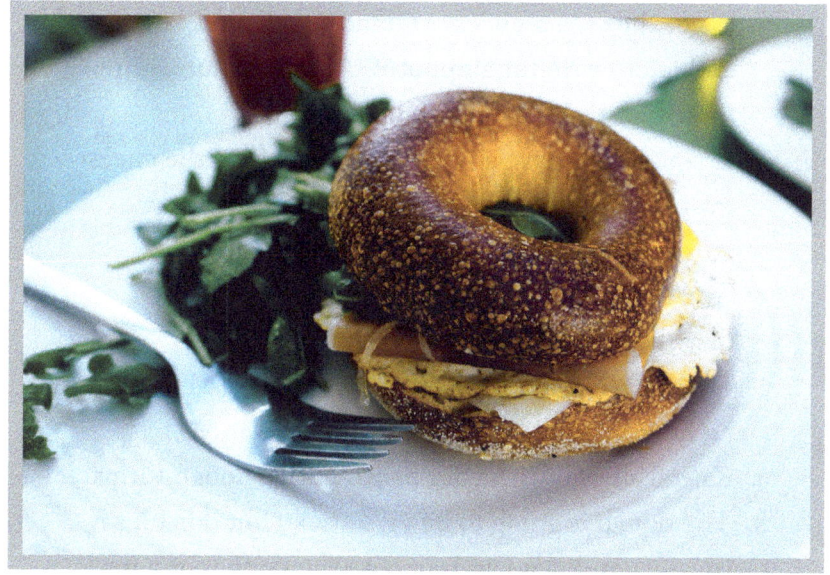

INGREDIENTS

- 145 g almond meal

- 1 Tbsp of Baked Powder
- Mozzarella: 283 g, grated
- 56 g Crème cheese
- 2 (L) L.

Topping alternative-sesame seeds

Powerful hint: A keto bagel baking mix is also available-tastes really good too!

PREPARATION

1. Set the oven to 200 °C and use baking paper to line the baking sheet up.
2. Blend the almond flour and baking powder together, then set aside.
3. Layer the cream cheese and mozzarella in a large bowl and microwave for 2 minutes. After a minute, remove briefly and stir again after 2 minutes.
4. If you do not have a microwave then heat the cheese over low heat on a double broiler on the burner, stirring continuously until it is fully melted.
5. Add the mixture of flour and eggs to the melted cheese.
6. Hint: Here you have to be fast, the cheese has to be hot.
7. Knead all well with your hands until a dough forms.
8. The dough is going to be very sticky but don't let it irritate you-knead and squeeze the dough for a few minutes with your fingers.
9. If the dough hardens before it is fully mixed, then for 15-20 seconds you can microwave it and heat it to

soften it. Wash your hands again before you start to knead the dough again.
10. Cut the dough into 6 sections and form each piece of dough into a long "sausage." Push the ends together- this is how the shape of the bagel is created.
11. Place pieces of the bagel batter onto the baking sheet. Sprinkle them over the bagels, and gently press them into the batter if you do want to use sesame seeds as a topping.
12. Bake 10-14 minutes at the bagels.

CINNAMON-APPLE BARS

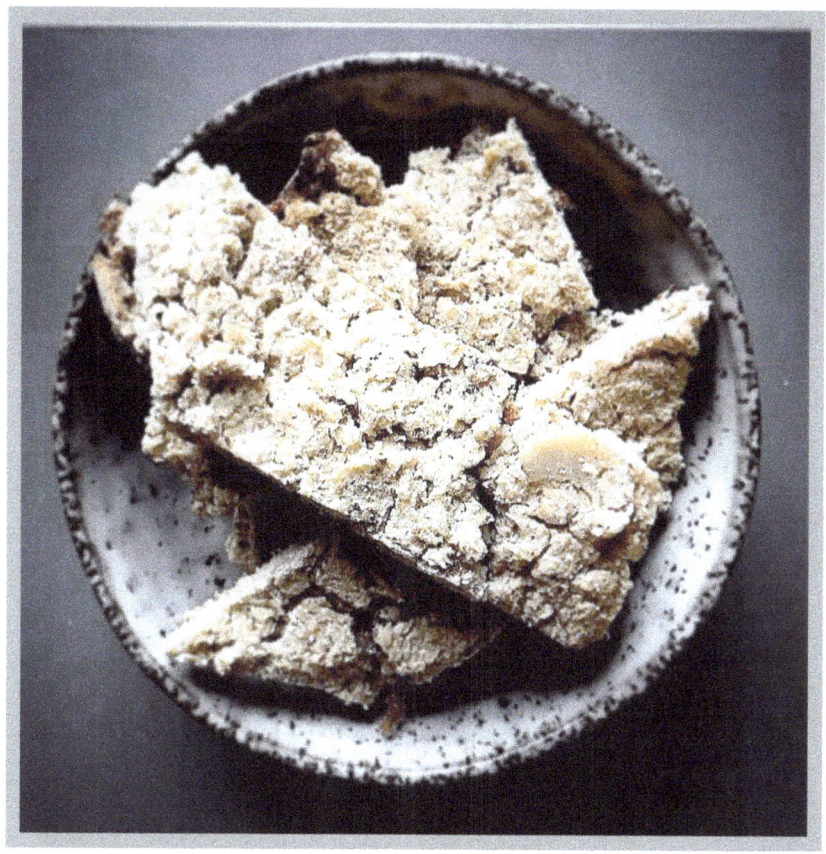

40 minutes

   300kcal

   Light

   6 serving

INGREDIENTS

- 4 Yeasts
- 1 Cup of pecan-trees
- 52 g cocoa fat

- ¼ tablespoon of frozen apples
- 2 Cinnamon Teaspoons
- 1 Vanilla Teaspoon Extract
- 10 Drops of stevia

PREPARATION

1. First, preheat the oven up to 180 ° C.

1. When you have no ground pecans then put the nuts in your blender and finely grind them.
2. In a mixing bowl, put in the eggs, coconut oil, vanilla, stevia, and cinnamon. All mix very thoroughly.

1. Add the dried apples and nuts (very small pieces) and stir all together.

1. Pour the batter into a saucepan and bake 25 minutes. The best way to do the wooden stick test is.

7
STAX FOR LOW CARB BREAKFAST

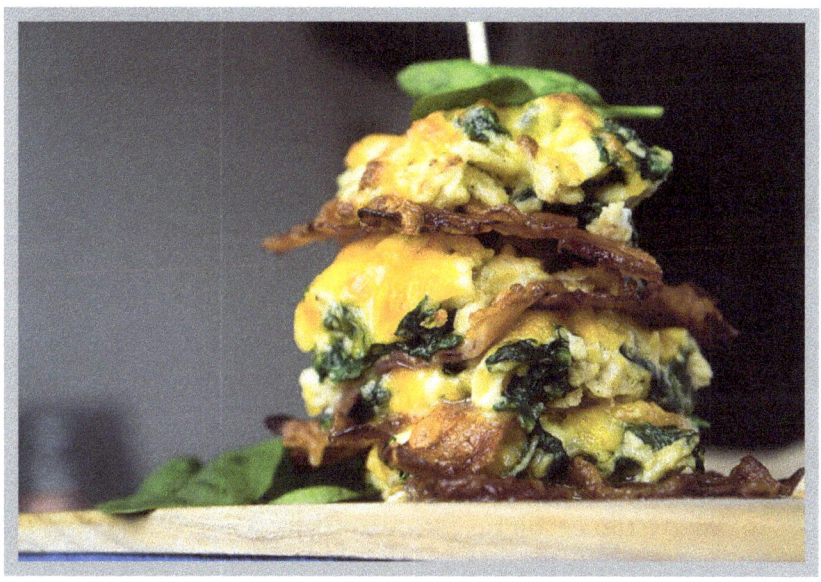

30 MINUTES
   230kcal
   Normal

4 serving

INGREDIENTS

- 10 Bacon Slices
- 2 cups of bacon fat
- 4 Spinach tassels
- 4 Grand Eggs
- 1/2 Cups of Cheese cheddar
- 2 Sheavy milk spoons
- Ms Dash table mix 1/4 of teaspoon
- 1/4 cubit kosher salt
- 1/4 tablespoon black chili pepper

PREPARATION

1. Preheat the oven until 400F.

1. Weave the bacon tie 5x5.

1. Place your cloth in the oven for 25 minutes. Start mixing your eggs and milk as it cooks.

1. Once tissue comes out of the oven, cut the tissue to extract the extra fat and put it on a paper towel.
2. Take 2-3 dc. Place the bacon fat in a saucepan with some spinach.
3. When the spinach is cooked add to your taste your eggs and season.
4. Place your eggs on top of the bacon tissue and stir.

1. Attach the cheese over the eggs and fry for 3-4 minutes in the oven.

1. Let them cool down for 5-10 minutes.

8
CHEESE FROSTING WITH BUTTER

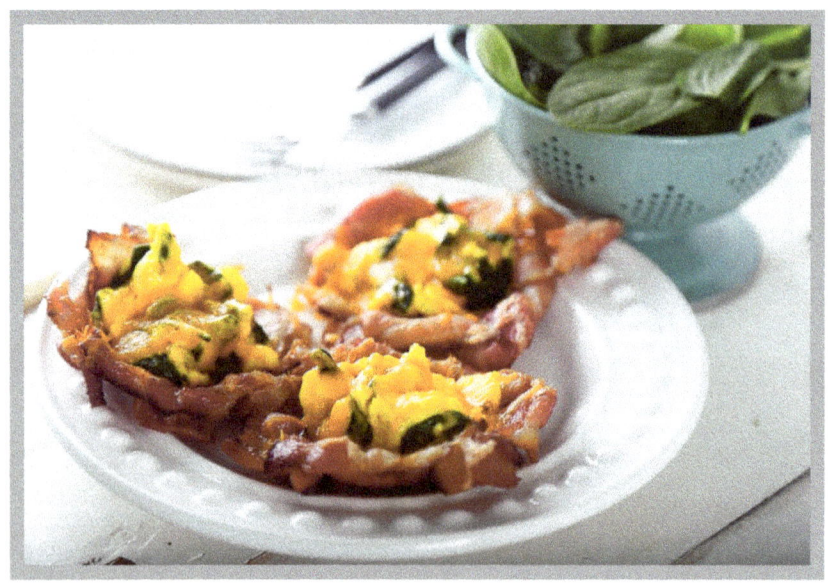

25 MINUTES
200kcal
Light

4 serving

INGREDIENTS

- 2 Spoonfuls of cream cheese
- 1 lbs of erythritol
- 1 Table litre of heavy cream
- 2 Batter Teaspoons left
- 1/4 Vanilla Extract Teaspoon
- 1/4 Cinnamon Teaspoon

PREPARATION

1. Mix all the ingredients which are dry.

1. Mix the mixture into the dry.

1. Put your batter on the waffle iron.

1. Add in the cream cheese filling while the waffle is

cooking.

1. The waffle fifth, then uniformly spread the cream cheese over half the waffle.

1. Place the waffle quarters unfrozen on top like a sandwich.

9
CRISPY BASKETS ON BACON

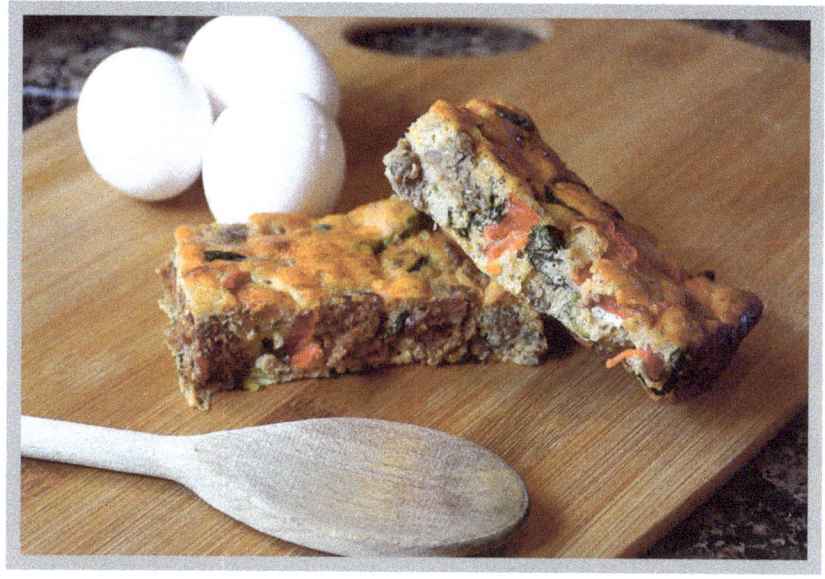

30 MINUTES
 311kcal
 Light

4 serving

INGREDIENTS

- 12 Bacon Slices
- 4 Grand Eggs
- 4 Spinach tassels
- Cheddar cheese: 2/3 cups
- 2 Sheavy milk spoons
- 1 spoonful of olive oil

- 1 Teaspoon potatoes

PREPARATION

1. Oven preheat to 350F.

1. Weave the bacon and cut quarters to pieces.

1. Flip a cupcake tray over, cover the four corners with foil and place the bacon tissue carefully on the foil.

1. Bake for another 50 minutes. Select, let cool for 10 minutes, and turn BROIL over to the oven.

1. Place two eggs in a cup, stir and add the milk.

1. Heat 1 lb of olive oil in a saucepan and cook the spinach. Attach some black pepper
2. When cooked the spinach add eggs and transform the heat to small. Food. Food.
3. Fill baskets of bacon with a mixture of eggs and spinach. Top on cheese.

1. Place in the oven and fry until it has a good crust in your milk. Entfer and serve.

THERE ARE: 325 calories, 26 g fats, 1.5 g net carbohydrate and 19.8 g protein per filled basket of bacon.

10
FRITTATA, EGG SAUSAGE

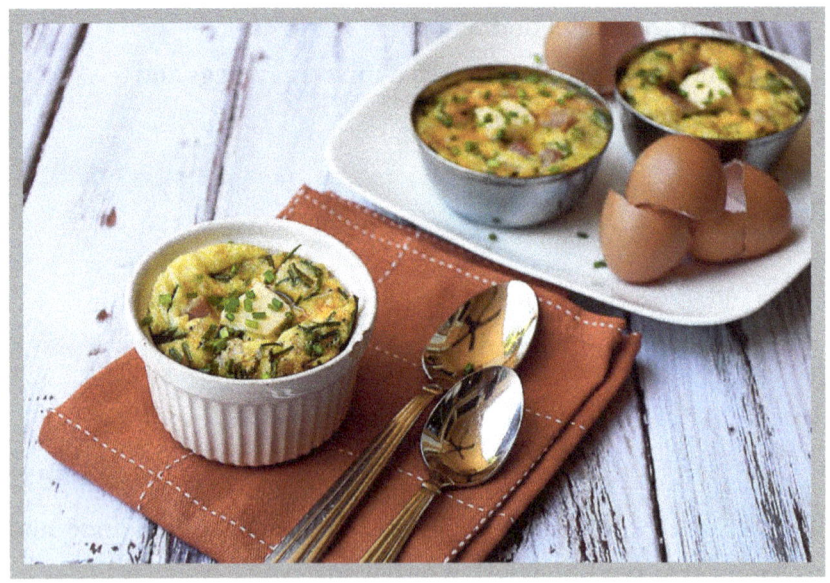

15 MINUTES
197kcal

Light
3 serving

INGREDIENTS

- Chorizo: ½ pound
- ½ Lb Italian Sausage
- Seven cups Spinach
- 2 Cheddar tassels
- 12 Large Eggs
- 8 Sheavy milk spoons
- ¾ cup of oignon
- 1 Half green pepper
- 1 spoonful of olive oil
- 1 Teaspoon Ail Dust

PREPARATION

1. Heat 1 tbsp of olive oil in a saucepan. Apply spinach, and allow to cook.

1. Crack 12 eggs in a large measuring cup or bowl, while the spinach is cooking. Apply 8 spoonfuls of cream and spices. Great blend.

1. Preheat the oven to 350 F as it cooks.

1. When the sausage has crumbled to your liking, add the spinach to the bowl and make sure to retain as much fat as possible in the pan.

1. Put the chopped onions and pepper in the saucepan and cook in the fat sausage. Bring it into the mixing bowl until finished.

1. Place the cheese in the tub, then gently blend.

1. Remove the eggs pounded, and blend well. Make sure everything's distributed evenly.

1. Place the mixture in a saucepan, wrap it in foil and butter.

1. Bake 45 minutes, at 350 degrees F. Once this is over, you will be able to drive a knife through that cleanly.

11
HAM, CHEDDAR AND CHIVES BLAST TOGETHE

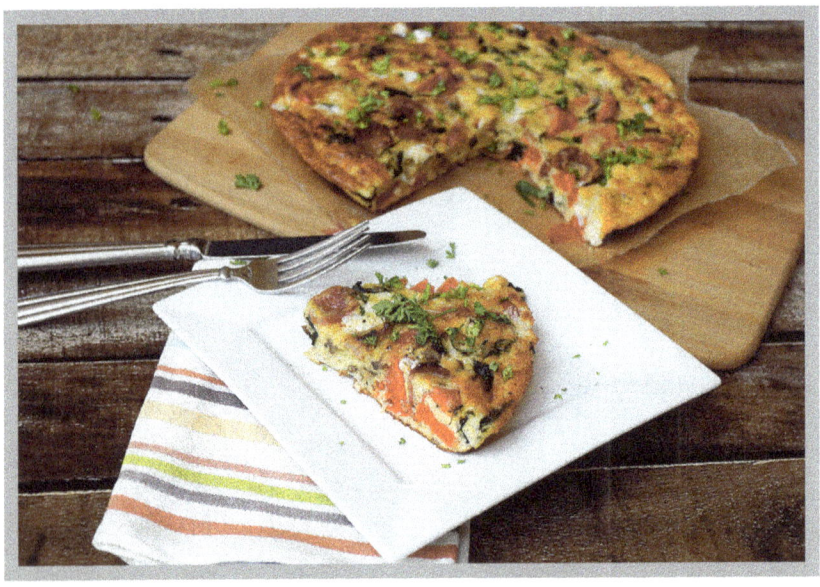

15 MINUTES
406kcal
Light

5 serving

INGREDIENTS

- 3 The olive oil spoon
- 1/2 Medium sized onion, chopped
- 1 1/2 teaspoon of captured garlic
- 6 Ounces steak ham, fried and chopped
- 1 Tablespoon butter for fattening casserole plates
- 6 Large Eggs
- 1 Piece of cheddar grilled cheese
- 1/2 Cup Strong Crème
- 2 Tablespoons of freshly chopped chives
- 1/2 cup of salt
- 1/4 cubit black pepper

PREPARATION

1. Oven preheat to 400F. Heat olive oil and add onions in a saucepan. When soft, add brown garlic.

1. Place all the ingredients in a bowl together and stir well. Divide the mixture into saucepan dishes and bake for 20 minutes.
2. Let it cool down a bit, and serve.

12
SPECK, ROTERPFEFFER, AND FRITTATA MOZZARELLA

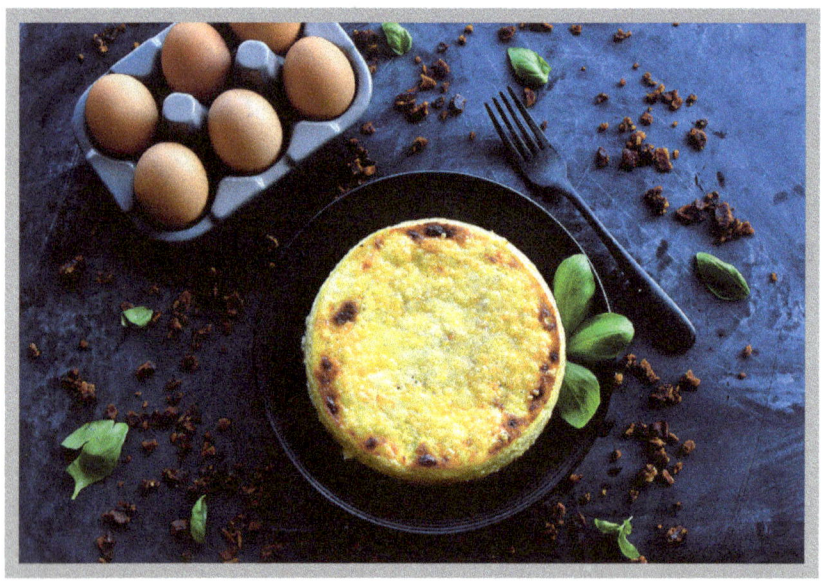

15 MINUTES
604kcal
Light

6 serving

INGREDIENTS

- 7 Bacon slices
- 1 litre of olive oil
- 4 Big champignon caps
- 2 Spoonfuls of fresh parsley
- ½ tablespoon of new basil
- 4 Ounces new, cubed mozzarella
- 2 Grated ounces of hard goat cheese
- 1 Half red pepper
- 8-9 Grand Eggs
- ¼ cup milk, strong
- ¼ cup Parmesan cheese, rubberised
- Great for salt and pepper

PREPARATION

1. Prepare your vegetables. Approximately cut basil, red pepper, mushroom and bacon. Mozzarella cube, and set aside. Oven preheat to 350F.

1. Place olive oil in a hot saucepan and wait for the first wisp of smoke. Upon the first wisp of smoke add your

bacon immediately.

1. Let cook the bacon until browned and then add red pepper. Leave the pepper to cook until soft in the bacon fat.

1. While the red peppers are cooking, add to a jar 9 eggs, 1/4 cup heavy cream, 1/4 cup parmesan cheese and fresh ground black pepper. Using a whisk to gently mix the eggs.

1. When red pepper is warm, add the mushrooms to the saucepan and stir well. Let the fat soak up in the mushrooms.

1. Add some fresh basil to pan and allow to cook for a moment, then sprinkle on top with cubed mozzarella cheese.

1. Pour eggs over this and use a spoon to raise the

ingredients at the bottom of the saucepan. You want all of the eggs in the pan to get under and around.

1. Rib 2 oz. Goat cheese over top and place for 6-8 minutes in the oven. Turn on the broiler then broil the top for another 4-6 minutes.

1. Take from the oven and pry the edges of the frittata away from the plate using your knife. Flip the frittata out of the saucepan until finished. Slice and then drink!

13
OVERNIGHT POMEGRANATE FLOUR AND FLAX SEEDS

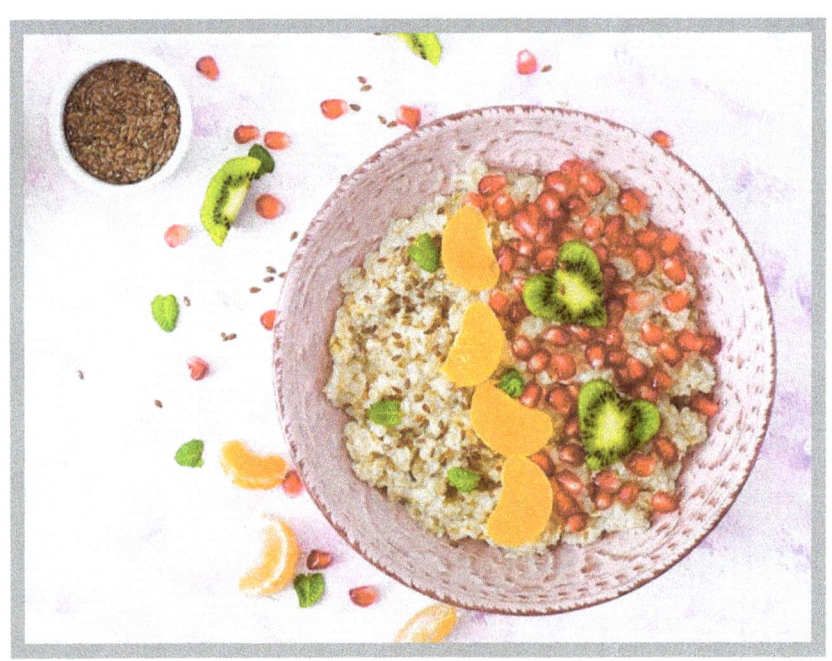

25 minutes
263kcal
Light
3 serving

KITCHEN EQUIPMENT
1 Table of jobs, 1 kitchen scale, 1 knife and 1 teaspoon.

INGREDIENTS

- 40 g Airbrush
- 120 ml organic soya beverage
- 30 g Grenade
- Kiwi: 30 g
- 30 g mandarin
- 1 Tbsp. Of flax seeds

PREPARATION

1. Put the oatmeal in a bowl or glass with the soy drink the night before, stir and soak overnight, hence the word oatmeal. • Oatmeal consumes fat, producing a thick paste.

1. In the morning, slice the kiwi, and cut it into bits. • scrape the tangerine. • Depending on how buttery you like it, you now can stir some liquid under the night oatmeal. • Spread the flax seeds over the night oats and then the pomegranate seeds, add the pieces of kiwi and mandarin. • Perfect for bringing with you

14
VITAL SALAD WITH YOGURT, VEGETABLES AND FLAX SEEDS

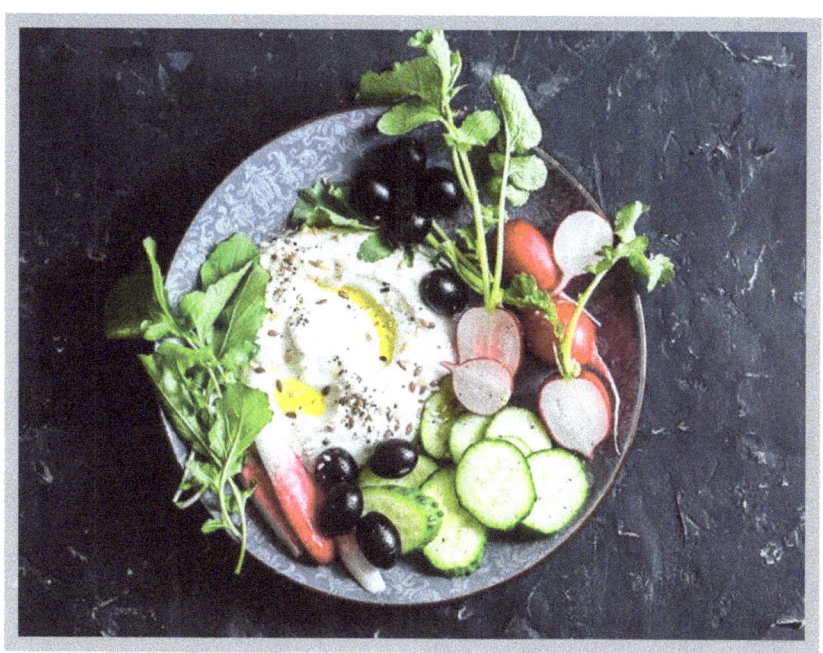

10 MINUTES

278kcal

Light

4 serving

KITCHEN-EQUIPMENT

1 Working plate,1 knife, 1 kitchen scale,1 press of garlic,1 teaspoon

INGREDIENTS

- 150 g Greek yogurt
- 100 g Cuckoo
- 100 g Crude Radishes
- 50 grams of Black Olives
- 1 A garlic clove
- Olive oil 1 Tsp.
- 1 Tbsp. Of flax seeds
- 1 Tsp Sesame Light
- Sea salt (salt fleur)
- Red Potatoes

PREPARATION

1. Position the yogurt in a bowl and stir in garlic (press the garlic and press the garlic) and olive oil. Add salt and pepper to yogurt.
2. Rinse and halve the radishes • chopped the cucumber into thinly sliced • Add the yogurt and serve with the flaxseed, sesame, cucumber, radish and olives.

15
EGGS SCRAMBLED IN LOW-CARB BREAD

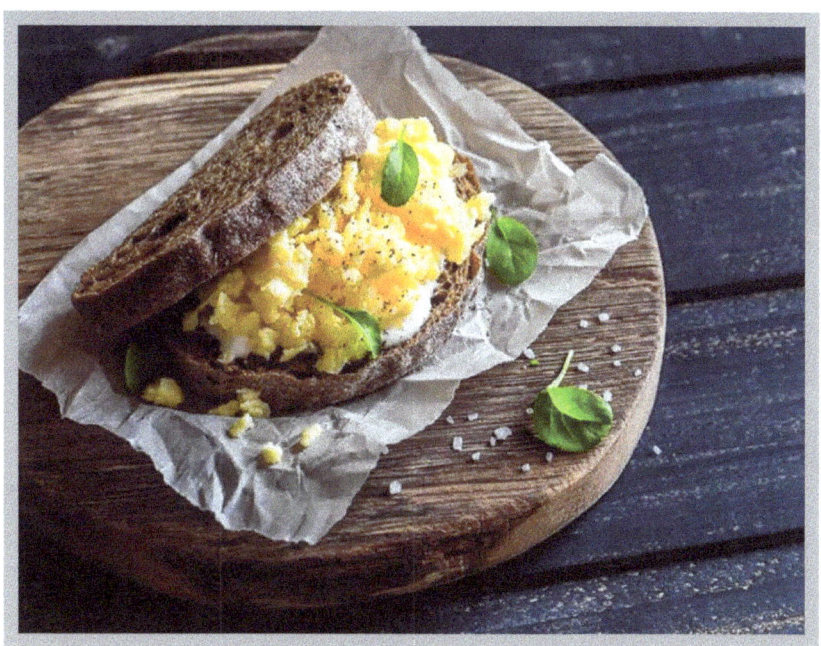

10 MINUTES

394kcal
Light
4 serving

KITCHEN-EQUIPMENT

1 panel,1 knife,1 bowl (stainless steel),1 whisk,1 grater,1 pan,1 spatula (wood),1 teaspoon.

INGREDIENTS

- 2 Cheese bread slices
- Size M. 2 Chickens.
- 20 g Granular Cheese
- 10 g Parmesan cheese
- Olive oil 1 Tsp.
- 1 Pinch of salt from the sea (fleur de sel)
- 1 Tablespoon black chili pepper
- 1 New Basil Stem

PREPARATION

1. In a cup, grate the parmesan and whisk the eggs, then season with salt and pepper.
2. In the pan heat the oil, add the eggs to the pan and allow to cool over medium heat.
3. Use the spatula to work through the egg mixture, so that it is cooked evenly.

4. Layer the bread with the granular cream cheese and layer the scrambled eggs over the end.
5. Clean and dry the basil, pluck the leaves and garnish the scrambled eggs.

16

VITAL MUESLI WITH CHIA, FRUIT, CHOCOLATE AND YOGHURT DROPS

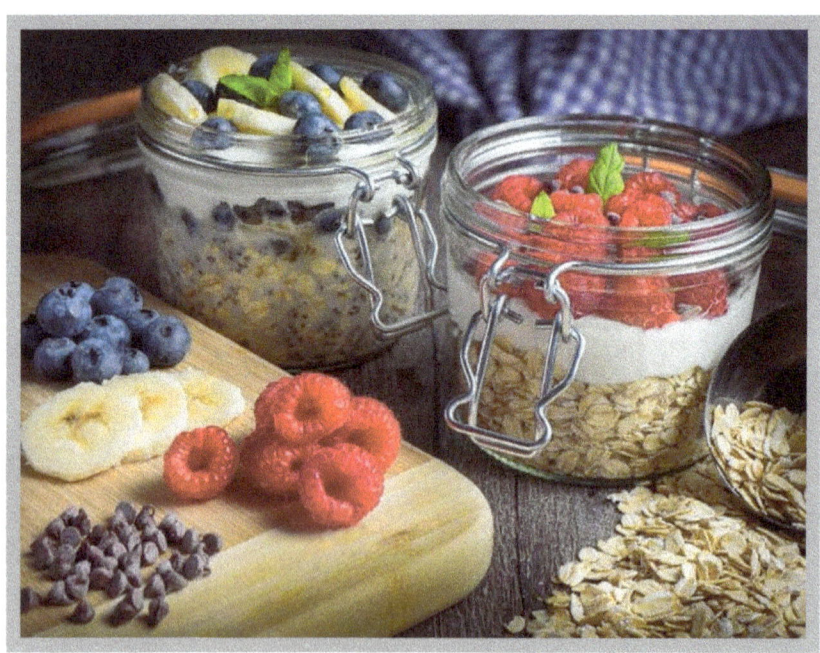

10 MINUTES

213kcal
Light
4 serving

KITCHEN-EQUIPMENT

1 Working plate, 1 knife, 1 kitchen strainer, 1 spoonful.

INGREDIENTS

- 50 g Airflour
- 1 Tbsp of Chia seeds
- Blueberries: 30 g
- 30 g Frambles
- 40 g Bananas
- 200 g yogurt
- 10 g Xucker chocolate drops 75% (chocolate with xylitol)

PREPARATION

1. Within a cup the chia seeds are mixed with water and left for approx. 20 minutes
2. Then mix 2 tablespoons of oatmeal under chia seeds (mix in a little more water if necessary)
3. Wash and drain the blueberries and raspberries.
4. Strip and cut into thin slices of banana.
5. When you work you will give free rein to your own

imagination.
6. We put the chia oatmeal mixture in a glass in our example, and serve it with yogurt, blueberries and bananas.
7. We balanced the remaining oatmeal in the second glass with yoghurt, raspberries and drops of chocolate.

17
STRAWBERRY CURD WITH WHEY, COCONUT FLAKES AND GOJI BERRIES

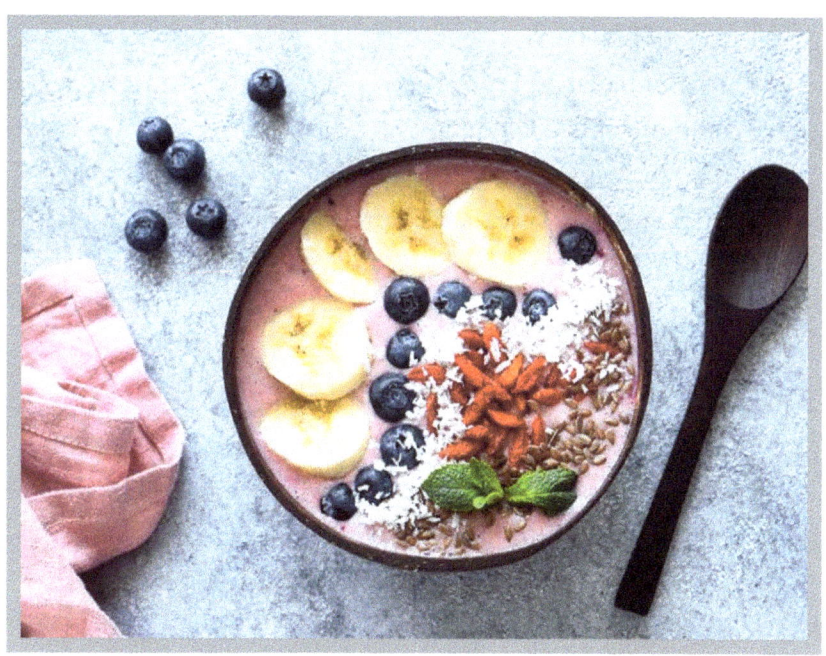

10 MINUTES

235kcal

Light

3 serving

KITCHEN-EQUIPMENT

1 Tablet,1 knife,1 kitchen scale,1 side blender.

INGREDINTS

- 150 g of curd,
- Lean 50 g of fresh or frozen strawberries
- 30 g of blueberries
- 40 g of banana
- 1 tsp of rubbed coconut
- 1 tsp of goji berries
- 1 tsp of Agave syrup as required 1 hand blender

PREPARATION

1. Place the strawberries and curd with the hand blender in a blender container, and puree. • Season the strawberry curd with agave syrup or other sweetener of your choosing, if you want.

1. Rinse and drain the blueberries • Cut and slice the banana • In a cup, put the strawberry curd, and add blueberries, banana slices, linseed, goji berries and coconut flakes.

18
LOW CARB AVOCADO MUFFINS

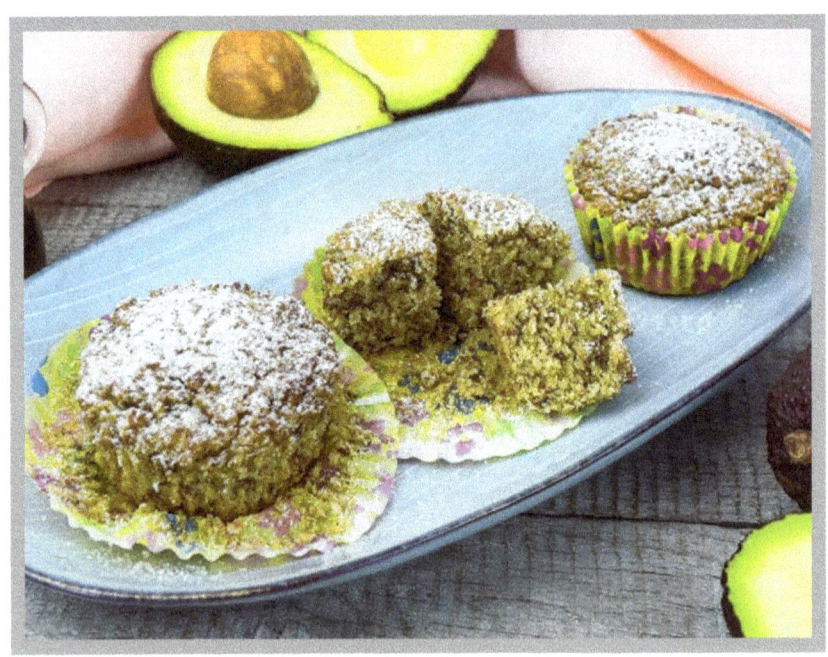

30 MINUTES

299 kcal
Light
1 serving

KITCHEN-EQUIPMENT

Set of 6: 1 mixing bowl, 1 hand mixer, 1 hand blender, 1 kitchen scale, 1 knife, 1 work plate, 1 table-litter, 1 muffin tin.

INGREDIENTS

- ½ New outrage at avocado
- ½ Crude Lime
- 2 Rough Eggs
- Avocado oil: 45 ml
- 100 g Basic xucker (Xylit FR)
- 100 grams of ground almonds
- 30 grams of coconut flour
- 10 G husk with psyllium
- Weinstein 0.5 bag of baking powder

PREPARATION

1. Break the eggs in a bowl • Add the avocado oil and xucker, and stir the electric hand mixer until creamy.
2. Halve the avocado and cut the heart off. Using a knife, scrape half the pulp and put it in a mixing bowl.
3. Attach the egg mixture with the ground almonds,

coconut flour, psyllium husk, and baking powder and blend in. • Line the 6-piece muffin tin with paper cases, and uniformly distribute the dough.

4. Bake the muffins on a medium shelf in a 160 °C preheated oven for around 20-25 minutes. • Remove the muffins and allow to cool. • Dust before serving, with a little powdered sugar.

19
PROTEIN AND APPLE PORRIDGE

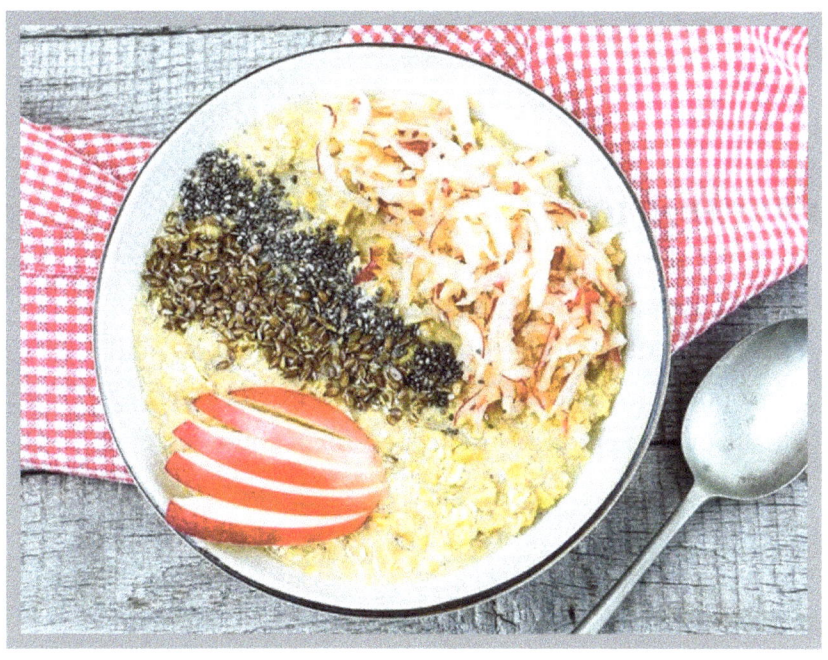

10 MINUTES

360kcal
Light
1 serving

KITCHEN-EQUIPMENT

1 Knife, 1 working plate, 1 grater, 1 spoonful.

INGREDIENTS

- 60 g Socas porridge protein Cinnamon apple
- 1 Apple
- 1 Tbsp of Chia seeds
- 1 Tablespoon of ground flax seeds

PREPARATION

1. Take water to a boil.
2. Place the porridge protein in a spoonful bowl and pour 120 ml heated water over it. Remove the porridge and allow to heat up for 3-5 minutes.

1. Meanwhile, wash and quarter the apple, and remove the core. Grate the pieces of apple with the grater and then add the chia and linseed to the porridge and serve wet.

20

BREAKFAST WITH PROTEIN LIKE SOY SEEDS, ALMONDS AND FIGS

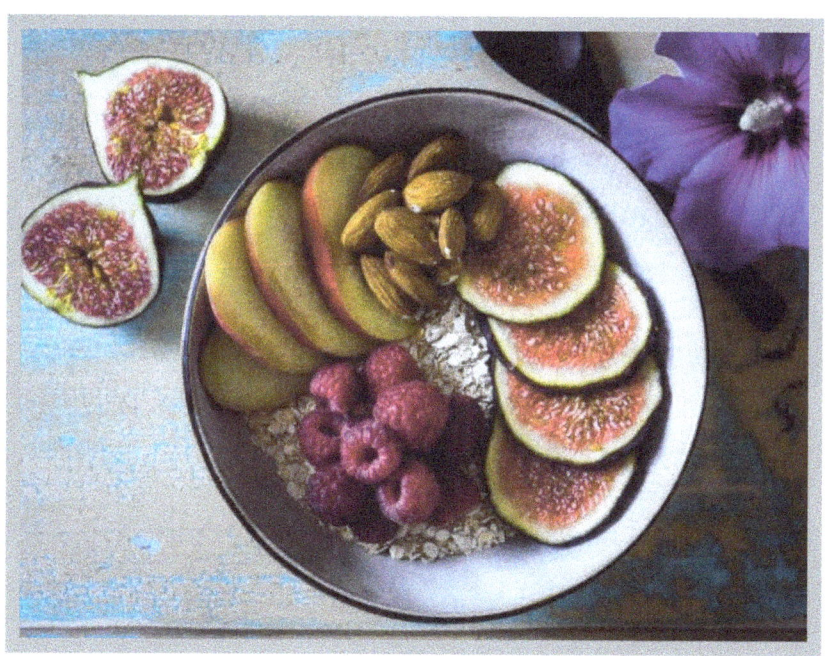

5 MINUTES

564kcal
Light
4 serving

KITCHEN-EQUIPMENT
1 Knife, 1 Tablet
INGREDIENTS

- 1 Pitcher
- 50 g Framboises
- 1 Ill.
- 30 g Mandarins
- Socas Protein Fine Flakes 65 g (de-oiled soy flakes)
- 250 g yoghurt

PREPARATION

1. Position fine soy flakes in a bowl for the breakfast. Rinse the peach, fig and raspberry and drain away. Cut peach in half, drop core and cut into slices. • The fig is sliced into slices.
2. Put the peach and fig slices on the soy flakes along with the raspberries. • Add the almonds and if you want, you can chop them roughly. Simply add the soy yogurt and mix.

Hint: Prepare the soy flakes with the soy yogurt for a meal, then add the fruit in small pieces

PROTEIN BARS WITH DATES AND SOYA FLAKES

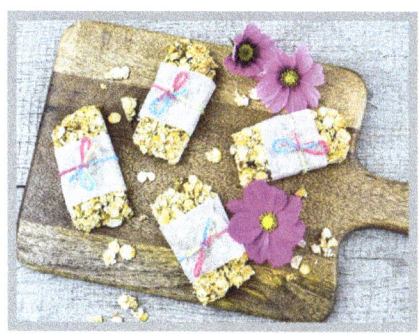

5 minutes
98 kcal
Light
8 serving

KITCHEN EQUIPMENT

1 knife, 1 work table, 1 bowl conduct ,1 Pound of peanut butter.

INGREDIENTS

- 100 g Socas protein flakes (soy flakes without oil)
- 50 g soy flakes without oil (soy flakes without oil),
- 20 g oil protein and vanilla ice cream
- 3 quotes

- 50 ml organic soy drink

PREPARATION

1. Position dates, chop and combine, and a bowl of flakes, protein powder, soy beverage and peanut butter if desired. • Knead the mixture and pour it into a baking sheet lined with baking paper.
2. Stretch the dough uniformly over around one quarter of the sheet and bake at a temperature of 175 °C (8-10 minutes) in a preheated oven. •
3. Attach the posts then to align the tibia and the ideal form of the pin. • Let the bar refrigerate and store securely.

21
FRUIT BOWL WITH APRICOTS, SOYA FLAKES AND FLAX SEEDS

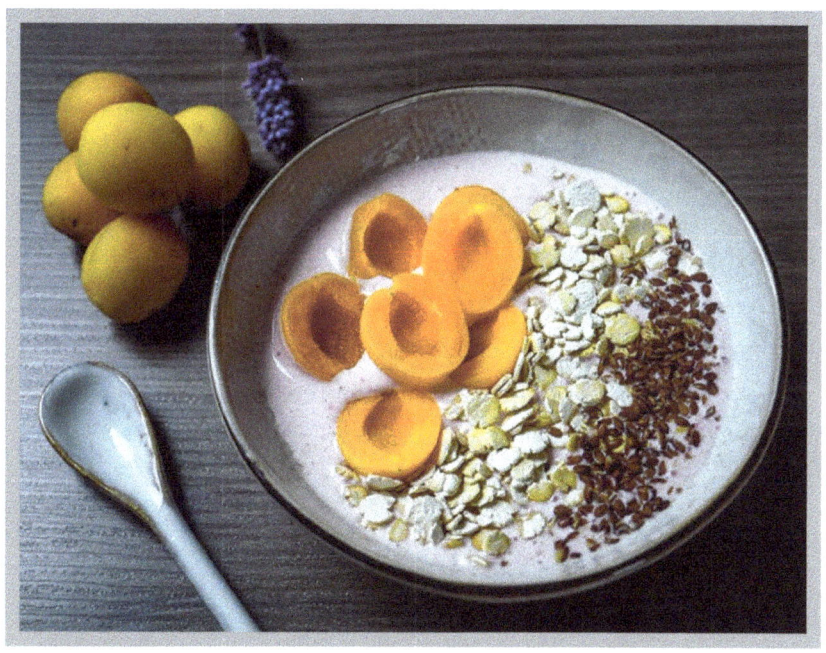

5 MINUTES

374 kcal
Light
1 serving

KITCHEN-EQUIPMENT

1 Hand mixer, 1 knife, 1 cup to weigh, 1 table to work.

INGREDIENTS

- 50 g Framboises
- 200 g of 3.5 per cent fat yogurt
- 3 Rough Apricots
- Protein flakes 25 g socas (soy flakes without oil)
- 15 g Field Flaxseed

PREPARATION

1. Position the raspberries and yogurt with the hand blender in a blender pot, and puree.
2. Wash and halve the apricots, then cut the heart.

22

ACAI SUPERFOODS BOWL WITH MUESLI, BLUEBERRIES AND COCONUT FLAKES

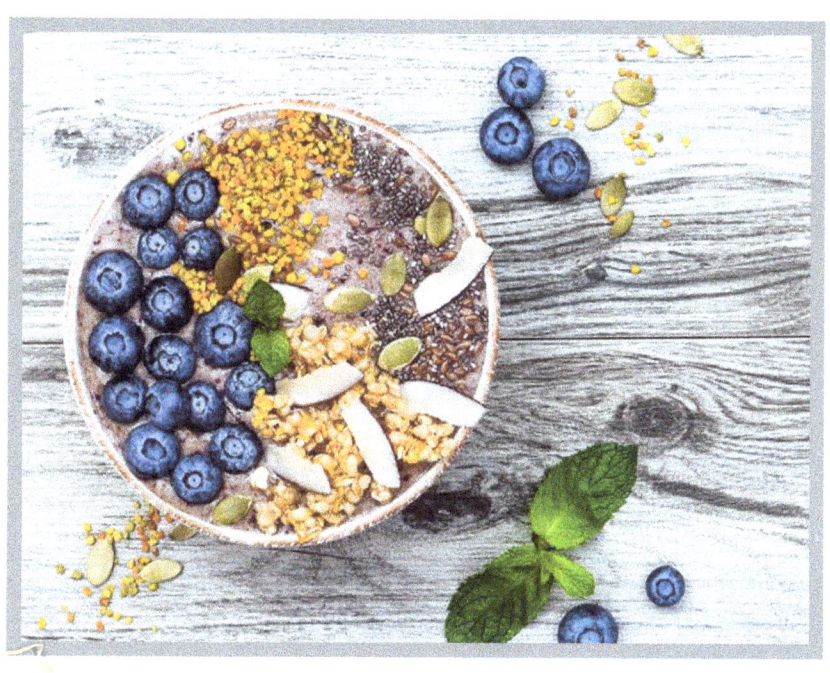

10 MINUTES

545 kcal

Light

1 serving

KITCHEN-EQUIPMENT

1 countertop, 1 kitchen scale, 1 cubicle, 1 tablespoon.

INSTRUCTIONS

- Greek yogurt: 250 g
- 1 Tbsp. Acai powder
- 1 Lightly greased tablespoon cocoa
- Blueberries: 40 g
- 1 Spoonful of Chia seeds
- 5 g Rasped coconut
- Poland 1 Teaspoon
- 1 Teaspoon of roasted pumpkin seeds
- 20 g Muesli coconut

PREPARATION

1. Agave syrup as required procedure blend the yogurt with the acai and cocoa powder.
2. soften the yoghurt and put it in a bowl with a little agave syrup.

3. Clean the blueberries and drain, then pour over the yoghurt.
4. Collect and serve the chia seeds, grated coconut, sticks, pumpkin seeds and muesli, and the bowl.

23
SUPERFOOD YOGURT, COCONUT AND NUTS

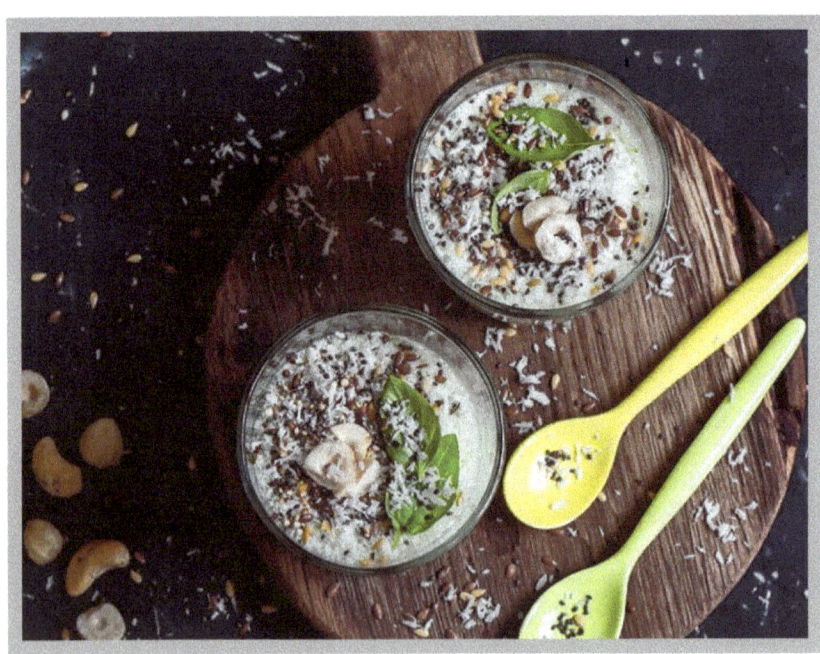

10 MINUTES

318 kcal

Light

2 serving

KITCHEN-EQUIPMENT

1 Table of jobs, 1 knife, 1 hand mixer, 1 kitchen scale, 1 salt, 1 cubicle.

INGREDIENTS

- 300g yogurt
- 1.5 percent fat
- 2 kiwi
- 2 flaxseed teaspoons
- 2 rubbed coconut teaspoons
- 2 chia seed teaspoons
- 1 sesame teaspoon
- 20 g cashews
- 20 g hazelnuts

PREPARATION

1. Put the yogurt and kiwi fruit in a blender jar and puree with the hand mixer
2. Put the kiwi yoghurt in two cups.
3. To kiwi yogurt add flax seeds, sesame seeds, coconut flakes and chia seeds.
4. Chop the cashews and hazelnuts thinly and add to kiwi yogurt.

24

EGG MUFFINS WITH HAM AND VEGETABLES

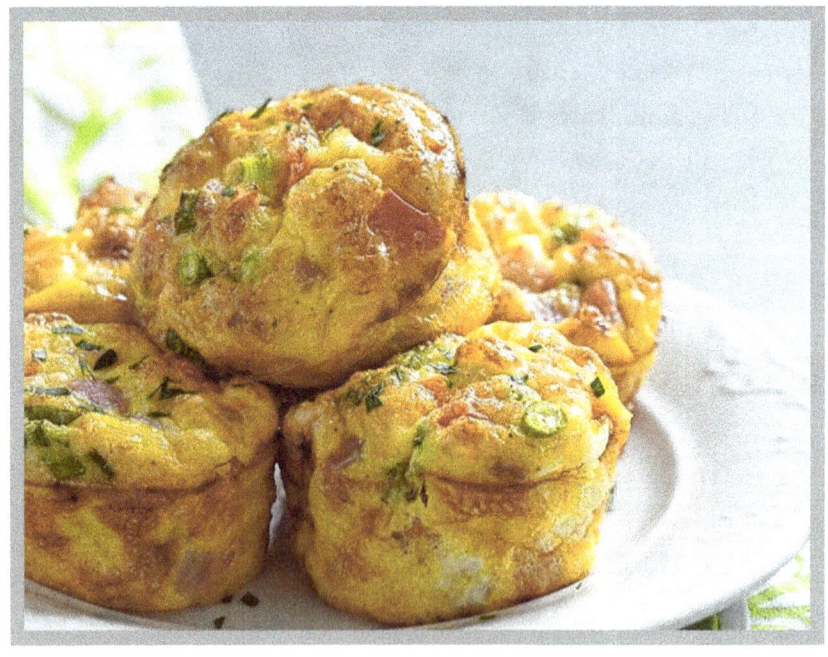

10 MINUTES

186 kcal
Light
6 serving

KITCHEN-EQUIPMENT

1 Table of job, 1 knife, 1 cup, 1 brush, 1 kitchen scale, 1 cloth of muffin, package of 6, 1 spoonful.

MATERIALS

- 6 eggs M.
- 2 Tablespoons of 30 per cent whipped cream
- 1 Pinch marine salt
- 1 Tablespoon black chili pepper
- 1 Sweet onion / s

- 80 g of fresh red potatoes
- 70 g Ham at Parma
- 2 Sticks of petrol
- 1 1 cup of olive oil
- Parmesan: 70 g

PREPARATION

1. Season with salt and pepper • Cut the tender onion

into rings

2. Cut the pepper into tiny bits •chopped the Parma ham into small cubes. Xclean the parsley and shake dry, then chop • Grate the Parmesan cheese • Brush the muffin boxes with oil and carefully pour mixture of the egg cream into the 6 boxes simply add the processed ingredients to the boxes and afterwards add the Parmesan cheese.

1. Position the muffin boxes in the preheated oven and bake at 175 ° C for about 20 minutes • afterward carefully remove the muffins from the pan and remove the edge of the pan with a knife if necessary • Season the muffins with salt and pepper again

25

BATIDO DE FRUTAS WITH YOGHURT, PINEAPPLE AND ORANGE

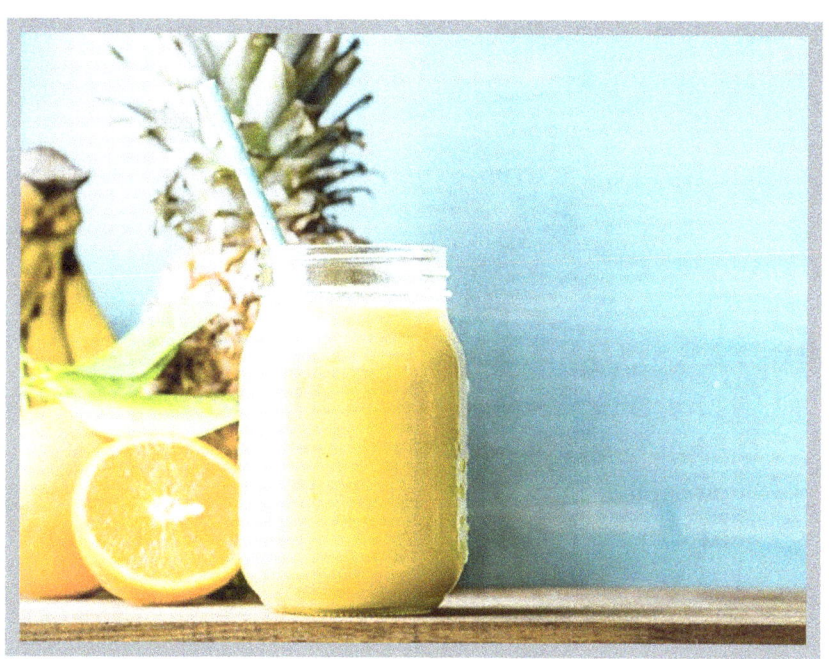

10 MINUTES

Light

2 serving

KITCHEN-EQUIPMENT

1 Panel, 1 knife, 1 mixer, 1 kitchen scale, 1 teaspoon

INGREDIENTS

- 200 g yogurt, 3.8 per cent natural
- 50 g Crude Pineapple
- 40 g Orange
- 50 g Bananas
- 50 ml of potable water as needed
- 1 Pressed teaspoon of fresh lemon juice
- 1 Tsp of agave syrup, as needed

PREPARATION

1. Extract and detach the rough middle part of the pineapple, then cut into pieces • Strip orange • Peel banana and cut coarse pieces.

1. Place the pineapple, peach, and banana into the

blender and puree with yogurt and sugar. • Season the fruit with lemon smoothie and agave syrup and put it into two glasses.

26
MANGO-GRANOLA

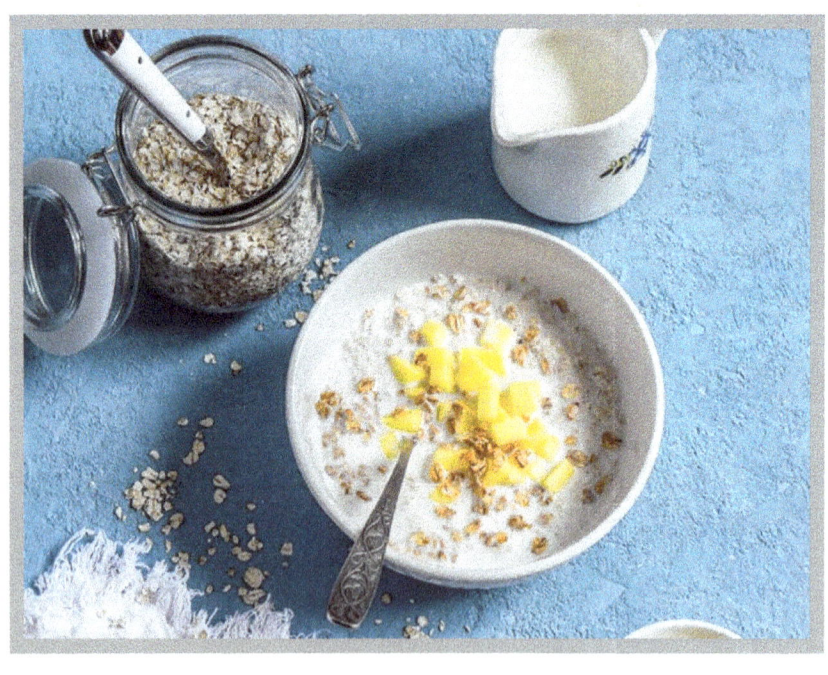

15 MINUTES

323 kcal
Light
1 serving

KITCHEN-EQUIPMENT

1 Table of jobs, 1 knife, 1 kitchen scale, 1 frying pan, 1 spoonful.

INGREDIENTS

- 20 g Hawthorn
- 20 g Split almonds
- 2 Cups of agave syrup
- 1 Pinch of cinnamon
- 30 g Hold
- 200 ml organic soya beverage

PREPARATION

1. Roast the oatmeal and the almonds gently in a fat-free pan, combine with the spatula several times. • Stir in the agave and cinnamon. Put the cereals on a large plate to cool down. • Cut the mango pulp into tiny bits, when doing so. • Place the mango muesli and soy drink in a cup, then serve.

27
PASTA LOW IN CARB WITH TOMATOES, COURGETTES AND BROCCOLI

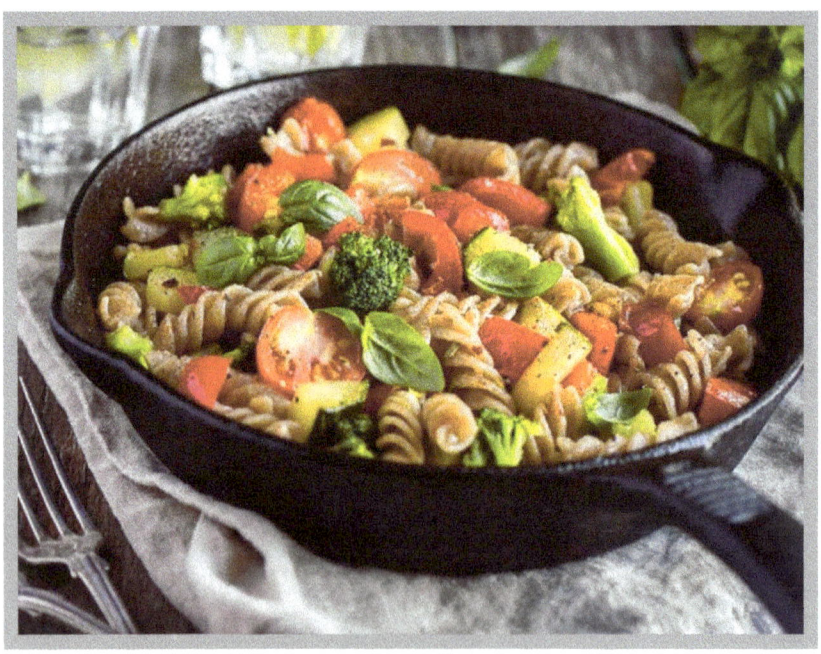

25 MINUTES

170kcal
Light
2 serving

KITCHEN-EQUIPMENT

1 pot, 1 strainer, 1 plate, 1 knife, 1 cup of measurement, 1 spatula (wood), 1 cubicle, 1 teaspoon.

INGREDIENTS

- 60 g fusilli low in carbohydrates-high pasta protein
- 80 g courgettes
- 10 Loved tomatoes
- 50 g Broccoli
- 50 g New red potatoes
- 1 Shallot
- 1 Knob
- 1 Tbsp of salt (salt fleur)
- 1 Pinch hot chili pepper
- Olive oil 1 Tsp.
- 1 Tbsp Paste Tomato
- 2 Fresh Basil Sticks

PREPARATION

1. Heat low carbohydrated pasta "al dente" in salted water. • Well rinse the vegetables and allow to drain. • Halve tomatoes with cherry. • Lengthwise quarter the zucchini, and cut into small strips.

2. Chop the broccoli florets from its stem, slashed into tiny pieces based on the size • Slice the bell pepper into thin slices • Peel the garlic and cut it into thin slices • Peel the shallot and dice finely.

1. Fry the cubes of garlic and shallot in oil saucepan. • Stir in the vegetables and fry properly. • Stir in the tomato paste and fry briefly.

1. Deglaze with a little pasta water on everything. • Then add enough water to the pasta until a sauce has enough liquid in the pan. •Let the pasta boil for a brief moment. Simply add the cooked low-carb noodles to and swirl through the vegetables in the pan. • Season with salt and pepper, cover with basil and serve.

28
SPINACH FRITTATA AND CREAMY GRANULAR CHEESE

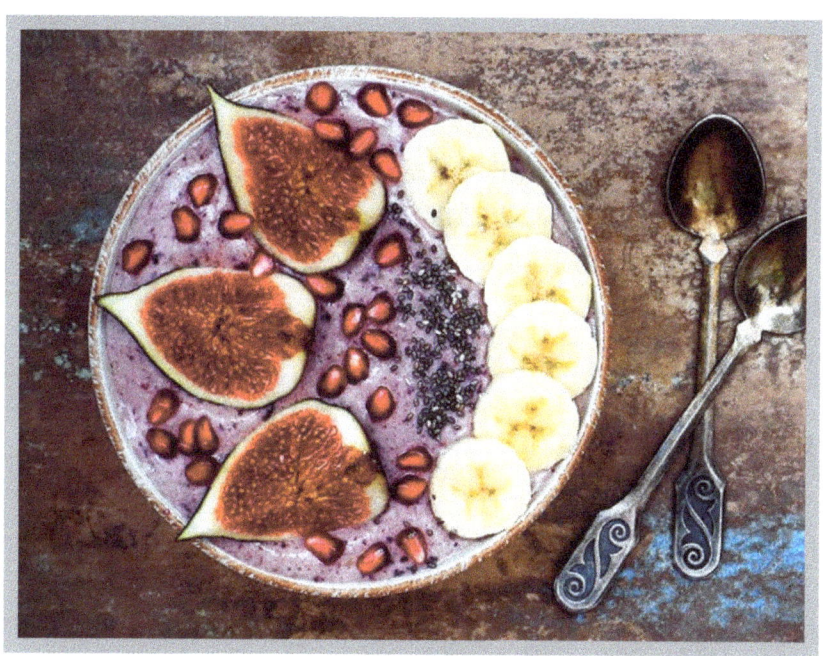

40 MINUTES

399kcal
Light
2 serving

KITCHEN-EQUIPMENT

1 table for work, 1 bowl (stainless steel), 1 brush, 1 centrifuge, 1 scale for the kitchen, 1 grater, 1 spoonful, 1 Tablet.

INGREDIENTS

- 4 The size of an egg
- M. 30 g Crude Spinach
- 3 Tablespoons of 30 percent whipped cream
- 50 g Parmesan cheese
- 100 g cream granular cheese, 20% fat 1 Tr
- 1 Pinch of salt from the sea (fleur de sel)
- 1 Tablespoon black chili pepper
- 1 1 cup of olive oil

PREPARATION

1. Rinse the spinach well, then drain. • Mix the eggs and whipped cream in a tub. • Stir in cream cheese and sauté with salt and pepper. • Mix it all up quickly again.
2. Heat the oil in the saucepan and add the mass of the egg. • Add the spinach leaves and let the mass of the

egg freeze over medium heat. • Apply the freshly grated Parmesan cheese over the mass of the eggs.
3. In the oven preheated to 180 ° C, place the frittata in the pan for 15-20 minutes. • And remove the finished frittata from the oven and cut it into pieces, sprinkle with a bit of freshly squeezed lemon juice and serve.

29
POWER-DRINK WITH ORANGES AND CARROTS

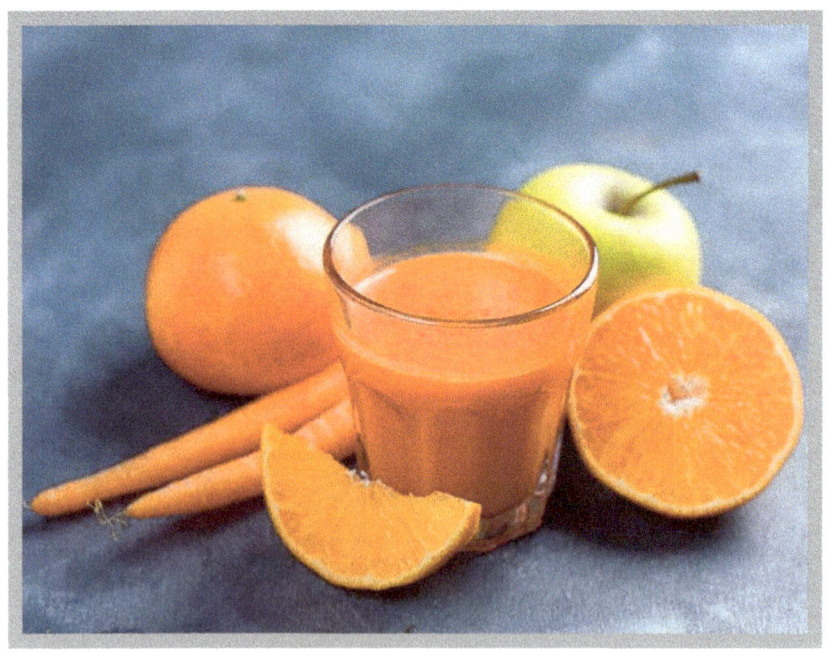

5 MINUTES

114 kcal

Light

1 serving

KITCHEN-EQUIPMENT

1 Hand mixer, 1 table to work, 1 knife.

INGREDIENTS

- 1 Small orange, new
- 1 Cartouche
- 50 g Apple Crude
- 1 g Rubbed Ginger
- 1 Pinch of cinnamon
- 100 ml of grip water

PREPARATION

1. Cut orange in half and squeeze • Peel the carrot and cut into pieces • Apple, wash, quarter and remove the kernel, then cut into pieces • Peel and chop ginger.
2. In a mixing bowl, place the orange, carrot, apple, ginger, and cinnamon juice together with the water and puree with the hand mixer. • Bring the orange-carrot energy drink into a bottle and serve.

30
GRANOLA WITH NUTS, ALMONDS AND YOGHURT

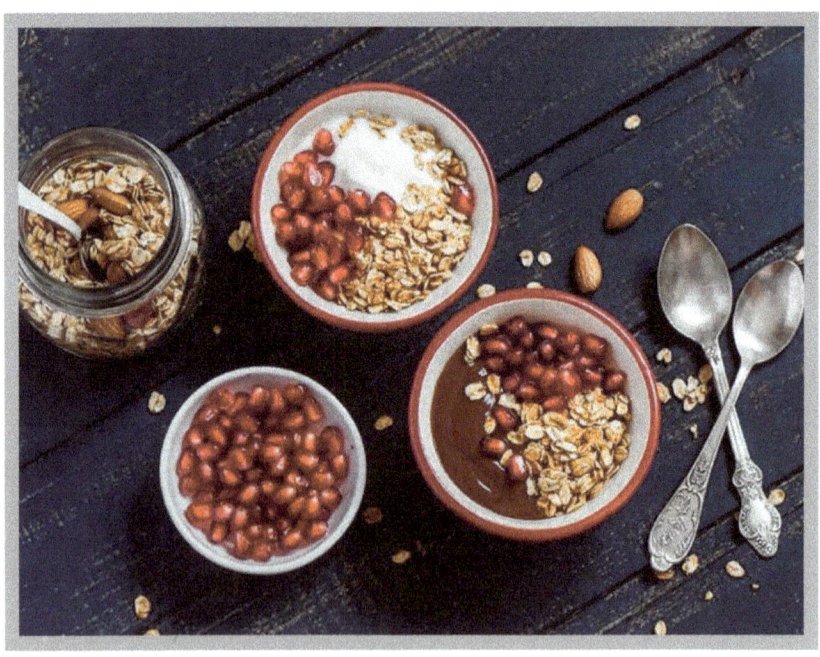

15 MINUTES

218 kcal
Light
2 serving

KITCHEN-EQUIPMENT

1 Working plate, 1 knife, 1 kitchen scale, 1 pan, 1 cup, 1 spoonful.

INGREDIENTS

- 60 g Grenade
- 200 g yogurt 1.5 fat per cent
- 1 Tsp cocoa, oiled lightly
- Cow 's 20 ml milk is 3.5 percent fat
- 60 g Flocks of organic oat
- 6 Mandarins
- Maple syrup according to need

PREPARATION

1. In a non-oiled saucepan, gently roast oatmeal, blend regularly with a wooden spoon. • Then remove the oatmeal from the pan and allow to cool.
2. In one shot, combine yogurt with milk and cocoa, season with maple syrup or another sweetener if needed. • Add a little more cocoa if you want it really chocolatey.

3. Fill in two bowls of almond yoghurt. • Cut the almonds finely and add them to the oatmeal yoghurt. • Carefully remove and add the pomegranate seeds from the bowl. • Stir it all up before eating.
4. Hint: If you prefer a muesli, pomegranate seeds, almonds and creamy or liquid yogurt for your breakfast, add a little milk or water and stir again.

www.ingramcontent.com/pod-product-compliance
Lightning Source LLC
Chambersburg PA
CBHW071117030426
42336CB00013BA/2126